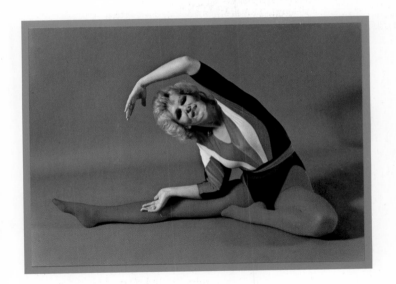

**Good
Health**

Fforbez

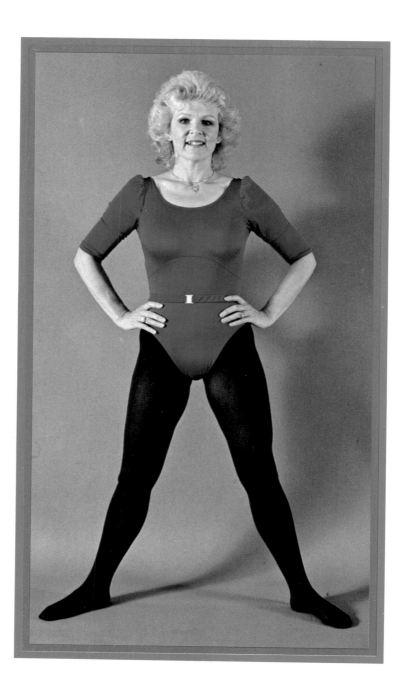

by **KAREEN ZEBROFF**

Controlling
HIP AND
TUMMY FAT
through
YOGACTIVITY

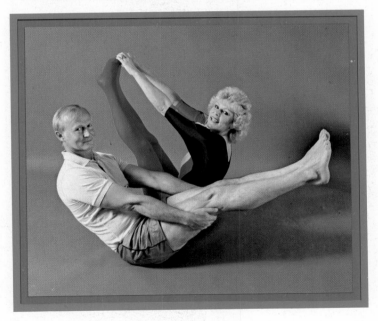

**Good
Health**

Fforbez

Canadian Catalogue
in Publication Data

Zebroff, Kareen, 1941 —
Controlling hip and tummy fat through Yogactivity
ISBN.   088976 · 071 · 3
1. Fat   2. Hips   3. Tummy   4. Yoga

The colour frames around each photo indicate:

_____ = for Women

_____ = for Men

_____ = for Women and Men

Copyright 1984
by Fforbez Publications Ltd.
Box 35340, Vancouver, B.C.

Photographs by   *Male Model*
Duncan McDougall   *Carl Floe*
Vancouver, B.C.   *B.S.A., M. Ed.*

Kareen's exercise suits by Renée Smith
of Pirouette Apparel

Edited by
Sylvie Zebroff

Printed in West Germany

Distributed by **Gordon Soules Book Publishers Ltd.**
1359 Ambleside Lane, West Vancouver, BC Canada V7T 2Y9
PMB 620, 1916 Pike Place #12, Seattle,WA 98101-1097, US
604-922-6588 Fax: 604-688-5442 E-mail: books@gordonsoules.com
Web site: http://www.gordonsoules.com

Table of Contents

DEDICATION
To all men and women who want to improve their lifequality through exercise

What This Book is all About

In writing this book it quickly became obvious that it would be a book with a difference. Over a decade ago, when I wrote the ABC of Yoga, I was one of the first Yoga-book authors to use an easy 'how-to' layout, rather than the more common prose style. Now I find myself once more writing a book that may very well be a first in Yoga.

After much study over the last fifteen years, I have come to the conclusion that the exciting answer to the baffling problem of fat-control lies in **combining** Yoga with a cardio-vascular (or aerobic) activity of your liking. For this reason, I have coined the new word 'Yogactivity'. This could be anything from swimming, bicycling and jogging to dancing, cross-country-skiing and trampoline-bouncing, followed by the gentle, stretching poses of Yoga. The 'aerobic' activity, however, must be done for a minimum of 12-15 minutes at 80% of maximum heartbeat if you are very fit, and for a minimum of 45-60 minutes at 70% of maximum heartbeat if you are a beginner, overweight or out-of-shape.

Unfortunately, the word 'aerobic' has become somewhat misleading these days. Actually, there is no such word in that context in the dictionary. It has only recently been coined from the Greek word 'aerobiosis' meaning literally "life in and by means or air or oxygen". An 'aerobic' type of activity might also be called a cardio-vascular, meaning "of the heart and blood vessels as a unified body system", activity. Of both these terms one could say that they generally refer to **constant, steady exercise** over a certain time period.

This time period will vary widely according to how fit you are and what you hope to achieve by your exercising. Only if you are very athletic indeed can you get away with exercising only for 12-15 minutes at 80% of maximum heartbeat, which you must carefully monitor by taking your pulse at regular intervals. However, if you are like most of the populace and have only recently developed an awareness of health and fitness, then you must start by working for longer periods of time at 70% of maximum heart-beat, again monitoring your pulse regularly. If that sounds horrific, don't despair, because if you are really out-of-shape your heart-beat could come up to 70% of maximum just by standing around bending your knees! Everybody's percentage lies at a different level of activity. Your fit neighbour's maximum may have to be a jog!

For most people a brisk walk will do the job. That is less impossible as you may at first presume. There was a time in my life when a quarter mile seemed like an odyssey. Now I have been doing four miles an hour for five years with my energetic neighbours, chatting all the while. All I had to do to accomplish this was to get up one hour earlier. For a sleepy-head like me that was a major change, but it has given me many unexpected added benefits. The orientals say that the energy of dawn is especially strong and that you can 'tank up' on it for extra vitality. I couldn't say, but I now love the fresh, fragrant air of the new day, even when it is raining and imagine that it does me a lot of good.

The benefits of such exercise are tremendous from a fat-loss point of view. You see, after you have exercised for about 45 minutes at 70% of maximum heart-beat, your thyroid kicks in and stays up for several hours afterward. If you then eat regular meals, followed by some mild exercise (a walk around the block, if you are at work, for instance) can keep the thyroid working all day. The thyroid gland is the weight regulator of the body — its hormone secretions control body metabolism. It also regulates the rate at which the body utilizes oxygen and the rate at which various other organs function. You can see how important it is to get the thyroid gland to work as efficiently as possible. You can easily tell just when it is that it has started kicking in: you will suddenly get a second wind and start to sweat. Keep up the exercise a little longer and then start to wind down. In the beginning it may take all of 45 minutes to get the thyroid going, but after some time this may happen sooner and you will be spending much less time at exercising to get the same beneficial effects. Since "metabolism" refers to that process in the body which transforms food and sets energy free — some of that released as heat — the thyroid plays a most important role in fat-control. A forty-five minute exercise session at 70% of maximum heart-beat in the morning is especially effective for weight-loss. At night, it is particularly beneficial for the health of the body. Kinetic energy (energy associated with motion) produced by the muscles, has a chance to release into the tissue and organs overnight for longlasting exercise benefits.

Our 'Yogactivity' program has been designed to help you lose over-all body-fat, since spot-reducing per se, has long been known to be virtually impossible. Only through losing fat generally (see Stop the Spread of the Middle article on page 7) can you flatten fat-laden muscle and reduce the layer of fat on top of it. When you then add the toning, firming and stretching movements of Yoga, you are indeed able to achieve a virtual spot-reducing effect. The 'Yogactivity' combination of exercising, therefore, can be **uniquely** beneficial in helping the individual lose fat. Actually, it may very well be the only way of getting rid of both 'side-bacon' and intramuscular fat. With patience and perseverance and a minimum of four work-outs a week, your whole body will become harder, tauter, smoother and firmer. The end-result may well be a wardrobe that is two to three sizes smaller, than when you started out six months or so earlier.

What Yoga is All About

The essence of physical Yoga practise is to bring out the natural beauty and strength of your body. Hatha Yoga is the best of all physical exercise — it relaxes, rejuvenates, tones, firms, energizes and beautifies. The 'art' of Yoga itself is 5,000 years old and is comprised of meditation, breathing techniques, hygiene, and physical exercise. Yoga exercises resulted from extensive observation of the stretching movements of jungle animals.

Their secret lies in stretching muscles slowly. Yoga exercises are designed carefully so as not to put strain upon the body. You move into each pose gently and slowly, holding it for as long as your own personal comfort permits, then release the position slowly and relax for as long as you deem necessary. Pent-up tension and stress are removed from the stiff muscles by these slow languid stretches. They give a new awareness to the body and make you feel 'good in your skin', as the French say. Yoga helps to bring you back to the centre of the self through its gentleness and calm.

Anyone of any age can start Yoga and immediately

benefit from its positive effects. No matter what your age, flexibility or state of health is, you can exercise safely and with success. Yoga is a highly individual and personally progressive activity. Your advancements are only comparable to yourself. It is vital that you realize your own capabilities and limitations, and that you gauge your exercises according to your own criteria, alone. You go as far as YOU can. Therefore, you are doing your best and who can ask for more.

With Yoga comes grace, balance, poise and a toned and supple body. Trouble areas such as chubby thighs, rounded tummies and thick waists are stretched and firmed back to their naturally lean and sleek shape.

Yoga also renews energy and strength to the body. Contrary to opinions on aging, the body **is** a renewable resource. The body is the first home we know and the only one we ever truly inhabit, therefore it is essential that we respect and preserve it in good, healthy condition. Yoga provides you with the means to do that.

For your greatest benefit I would suggest that your exercising follow these steps:

1. Warm-up for three minutes as suggested on page .
2. a) Do a cardio-vascular activity (as described on p.) for 12 to 45 minutes. I like the stair-stepping, rope-jumping and dancing to rock music or mini-trampoline bouncing best.

   b) Extremely important: take your pulse frequently for six seconds during the constant, panting activity. Multiply by ten to get the heart beats per minute. This is the most accurate way since heart beat drops dramatically within 45 seconds. It is your safety net for not over-exercising, which would have a very negative metabolic effect on your muscles of which the heart is one.
3. Do the Yoga poses to cool you down. Stretching and firming the muscles changes the squat, fat-laden shape back to long and lean.

4. Have a shower to wash off dead cells and sweat and toxins as the skin may reabsorb some of these if left on too long.
5. (Note for the considerably overweight)
   Gentle exercise over long periods of time will be best for you. Keep taking your heart-rate. You may have to start with a very slow walk and gradually work up to chair-stepping. As long as your heart-rate is working within 70 to 80% of its maximum you are changing your muscle metabolism back to its original lean muscle mass. It is virtually your only way to take fat off permanently.

As in Yoga, you are doing excellently if you are doing your best, no matter what others are doing. If they are fitter than you they have to do more strenuous activity than you. All you may be able to do is lift your heels to get the heart-rate up.

If the little lazy saboteur within all of us is tempted to quit because you are not losing weight fast enough, remind yourself that your measurements are going to change. Learn to rely on how 'you feel in your skin' and give yourself at least six months to lose centimeters off your body. After all, crash diets and sporadic exercising results in only one person out of 200 keeping the weight off permanently.

Fit and Flat Through Yogactivity

As we get a little older and more out of shape, we start to spread in the middle. In the men, it usually takes the form of a bulging upper tummy that slowly takes on the proportions of a soft lumpy beach ball, forcing the man to drop his belt-level lower and lower.

In the woman, fat is accummulated in a pecise order: first on the back of the thighs, then the sides of the thighs, then the tummy and the midriff and finally the arms and the chin. When she diets, the woman loses fat in exactly the reverse order, starting with the chin. The legs will be the last to lose which explains the hip bulge so common to women. They simply never get to those areas, in their efforts with weight loss, as they become tired of the constant dieting. What they should be doing instead is constant exercise, in a balanced combination of Yoga and cardiovascular exercise — Yogactivity.

Unhappily, women have 30% more body fat than men. However, men have 20% more muscle than women and fat invades the muscles first. So, man's body fat is often more hidden than woman's. This is why it would be more accurate to say that someone is over-fat, rather than overweight. A man may not look it for five years of inactivity and overeating, but when his muscles have finally become saturated with fat, and the fat 'spills over' into surrounding tissue, and shows under the skin (subcutaneous fat), only then will he suddenly look pudgy and out of shape. He will be bewildered, because he has not recently done anything to deserve this onslaught, but his story really goes back five years. It took the muscles that long to get 'marbled' (a process that makes for excellent steaks in beef).

If you want to be absolutely trim and firm all over your body, then it is important to keep the percentage of body fat down to 15% for men and 22 - 23% for women. However, most overweight people (by the time you become overweight you have already been over-fat for some time) who are not fit, have body fat percentages of 23% to 80%. As you can see, muscles atrophied from disuse can be replaced by fat through inactivity (the footballer gone to seed), but the process can be reversed through EXERCISE, in a peculiar way. No exercise alone will help you to get rid of flab, you must also diet to get the weight down. But to KEEP it down and to lose ugly rings of fat, you must combine 2 types of exercise:

a) 12 to 45 minutes at 70-80% of maximum heart beat **and**

b) the gentle Yoga.

The **constant,** oxygenating (aerobic) exercises are necessary to exercise your cardiovascular system and to help you to get the fat out of the muscles.

But let me emphasize that it is the pace that is important here, not the speed. You bring your heart beat up to 80% of maximum and keep it there at a steady rate for the required time of 12-15 minutes, only if you are very fit. A beginner should exercise for 45-60 minutes up to 70% of maximum heart-beat, until such a time that he begins to perspire and gets his second wind.

The Yoga is absolutely necessary to stretch the fat-laden, squat muscles back into their long, lean shape. Also, particularily for the very overweight, it has been found that mild exercise, such as Yoga, done over longer periods of time burns a higher percentage of fat than sporadic bursts which burn mainly glucose. Together, however, these two forms of exercise will give you a superbly firm and sleek look.

Fat is 'general' fat, not local or specific. The body stores it wherever it finds the room. This is genetically determined by your body type. As I have often said before, you do not inherit **that** you are fat, only **where** you are fat. There is no such thing as tummy fat or hip fat. The body draws on its fat as you would draw money out of a general bank account — for all purposes.

However, if you have too high a body-fat percentage generally (and 98% of the population does), it will mean that all your muscles have turned from beautiful long, and slinky tissue, into short, bulky things. If you also happen to have layers of fat on top of fatty muscle, **then** you look bulgy. It is for this reason that we are concentrating our efforts on the hips, waist and abdominal muscles in this book. That is where most fat accummulates when the muscles are totally saturated.

A gradual diet plan like Weight Watchers, in which you eat a minimum of 1,200 calories and lose no more than one to two pounds a week will help you to get rid of some of the layer of fat under the skin. To burn the general fat, including the fat in the muscles, you need to do cardio-vascular exercises such as:

running-in-place	cross-country skiing
very fast walking	roller skating
swimming	ice skating
rope-jumping	chair-stepping
bicycling	mini-trampoline bouncing
dancing	rowing

or anything that raises the heart beat 70-80% of its maximum ability for a minimum of 12 to 45 minutes (see Do's and Don'ts on how to take your pulse). Personally, I do not approve of jogging as more and more evidence comes in, indicating that it may have several side-effects, especially for women.

Since spot-reducing of subcutaneous fat is virtually impossible, you must concentrate on exercising the muscle underneath. Manipulating the offending area is useless. I know. For years I had a stomach whose muscles were rock-hard from all the Yoga, but on top of them sat a persistent little roll of fat, that no amount of pummelling and rocking-and-rolling-over would remove. Many a yoga teacher had exactly the same problem. However, we were reluctant to lose weight beyond a certain point, because we started to look gaunt and haggard in the face. Now, after much study, I know why I had pockets of fat on my otherwise trim body and why weight loss made me look ill.

When you lose weight too fast on a diet, you lose muscle along with the subcutaneous fat. However you will lose the fat in the muscle only at the very last, under extreme starvation conditions. When you diet rigorously you also lessen lean muscle mass. In a recent study in Germany, healthy subjects were asked to fast until they had lost 20 pounds. Of these, seventeen pounds were protein-loss and only three pounds were fat-loss. In other words, the body was virtually cannibalizing itself. Therefore, it may be a good idea to get fit before going on a diet, because an exercised body responds with less muscle loss to the stresses of dieting than an out-of-shape one.

Experts on weight have been puzzled in the last few years by fat people who are on strict, supervised starvation diets and still gain. Contrary to popular opinion, fat people do not necessarily eat more than their slimmer friends. It is true that they do exercise less, but everyone knows of some enviable slim individual who can eat all he wants and who never exercises, either. Dieting by itself burns both muscle and fat and can only lead to dehabilitation and fatigue. Obviously, then, permanent fat loss is neither due to diet alone, nor to exercise alone, but to a combination of the two. We know now that more than 99½% of all the people who lose weight eventually gain it back and MORE! Why?

The reason is body chemistry. Slim people's bodies efficiently use up 100% of their calorie intake, whereas the body metabolism of the overweight uses up only 90% and turns the other 10% into fat. Unfortunately the fat person is very efficient in making and storing fat, but not in burning it. These people have a fat person's chemistry. The fatter we become, the more our bodies change their metabolism in order to build up more fat, rather than burning it off.

Muscle metabolism is too complicated a process to detail here. Let it suffice to say that only muscle cells have certain, specific enzymes that are capable of burning up huge amounts of calories in a very short time period. Ninety percent of all the calories burnt in the body are burned by muscles. It follows that when we use our muscles during exercise, we are increasing our calorie output (by up to 50-fold). Exercise also produces greater numbers of these enzymes. Therefore the fitter we become, the more we can change our muscle metabolism to eat more without getting fat.

Exercise makes more enzymes. These help the muscles to use the fat for more energy. Therefore, when you exercise you use up fat. It's that simple. And that complicated. Contrary to what some diet books say, fat is not hard to lose. All you have to do is exercise and watch what you eat and how much. And as you work out, keep telling yourself that you are making lots of fat-chomping little enzymes.

Some of the reasons why some people are slim and stay that way is that they eat only when they are hungry, they eat little and they move around more than fat people. They usually exercise subconsciously. That is to say, they fidget, they bounce around, they are always on their feet, they run rather than walk across the room and they are the first to get up to fetch something. In other words, they MOVE. This gives us an important clue.

In order to lose weight on a certain part of the body, IT IS NECESSARY TO EXERCISE THE WHOLE BODY. Paradoxical as it may sound, in order for you to get rid of bulges around the middle you must exercise the legs most! The reason for this is that they are the largest muscles in the body and therefore considerably more calories are used in exercising them than in exercising a smaller muscle. That is to say, when you exercise large muscles the body derives its energy for doing so by withdrawing fat from its all-over-body and subcutaneous stores. Hence the all-important leg and buttocks exercises. Generally speaking, the more you get your muscles into shape, the more the body turns food into energy, rather than converting it into fat.

In order to get rid of the 'side-bacon' in your body you must get rid of your dependence on your bathroom scale. It is entirely possible for someone to drop from a size 12 to a size 8 with our exercise plan and lose nothing, or even gain a little! When the fat is lost, first from subcutaneous layers and finally from muscle-fat, your shape will change from bulky to long, smooth and lean. This explains why people are the same weight as you but look so much slimmer. You must remember that even though your weight has stayed constant, the fat in the muscle has been replaced by muscle mass and muscle is much heavier than fat. So, you have lost a lot of fat, although your weight stays the same, because the heavy muscle took the fat's place. Only your clothes and a measuring tape will tell the tale. No scale can measure fat-loss! When your body fat percentage becomes considerably lower, you become immeasurably healthier, sleeker and fitter. All it takes is active exercising and the gentle art of Yoga — that's Yogactivity.

Heart Rate

As muscles work harder they demand more oxygen. Therefore, when you exercise the muscles your heart must beat faster. The harder the exercising, the higher the heart rate.

Each heart, male or female, has a maximum rate determined by age. This means that the pulse will not exceed this maximum rate no matter how rigorous the exercise. This maximum varies according to age. Young people of 20 have a rate of 200 beats per minute. As one grows older the maximum rate is lowered. No matter which sex or in what state of physical fitness you are in, this maximum rate remains constant with your age. To find out your own personal maximum heart rate subtract your age from 220.

E.g. My age is 42. My **maximum** rate should be 220 - 42 = 178. I must never exercise at that rate, however! That is much too strenuous. I must come down to 80% of maximum. If I consult the following table I can see that my heartbeat should never exceed 146. Neither should it be much less for the 12 minutes of aerobic exercise. (My maximum rate is at 80%, rather than 70%, because I am very fit and athletic.)

For everyday exercise to be efficient, we should be working hard enough to raise our heart rates up to but no further than 80% of maximum. (To find out your 80% maximum level, please consult the following chart).

Age	Maximum	70%	or 80% of Maximum (only if very athletic)
65+	150	105	120
60	160	112	128
55	171	120	137
50	175	122	140
45	179	125	143
40	182	127	146
38	184	129	147
36	186	130	149
34	187	131	150
32	189	132	151
30	190	133	152
28	192	134	154
26	194	136	155
24	196	137	157
22	198	139	158
20	200	140	160

Never push or slow yourself to exercise at another person's rate. What may be an 80% maximum for one individual is another person's 100% maximum and vice versa.

Men and women should not be advised to exercise together unless the man is older than the woman. This is due to the fact that men have 20% more muscle-mass than women and 30% less fat. Therefore the male requires more physical exertion to achieve his maximum than a woman, and women can be over-exercised when attempting to keep up the pace. When muscles are overexercised they not only hurt but also begin to burn glucose rather than fat. Women have a **resting** heartbeat of 80 and men of 72, by the way. Some people, however, have very low resting heartbeats, and these individuals should exercise at a maximum 2-3 places above the maximum for their age on our chart. E.g. My husband Peter has a low resting beat and at age 49 need not work up to 122 beats but only 112.

In order to find out if you are adhering to your 80% maximum pulse rate, exercise steadily for 2 minutes or so and then take your pulse for 6 seconds and multiply by 10 to get your beats per minute. If the pulse is below 80% exercise heart rate you aren't working hard enough. If the rate is too high then slow down slightly. REMEMBER, THAT SOME PEOPLE ARE WORKING UP TO MAXIMUM JUST BY LIFTING ONLY THEIR HEELS WHILE OTHERS, FITTER OR YOUNGER ONES, NEED TO RUN IN PLACE VIGOROUSLY TO GET THE SAME EFFECT.

Here are some tips on taking your pulse. Be sure to have a watch or a clock with a second hand nearby. You will find your pulse on the thumb side of your wrist. If you can't find your pulse easily, then try placing your fingertips against the side of your neck and one of your fingers will pick up the pulse. It is a good idea not to take your pulse with your thumb as it has a pulse of its own and the count may be doubled or distorted.

Be sure to check your 70% (or training) rate often, since after several weeks of similar exercise you may need to increase your exertion to maintain the training maximum. It is also equally important not to push the rate over the training pulse. Everyone should, of course, **check with** his **doctor before starting** routinely on any exercise or diet regime. This is especially important if you are overweight, over forty or have a chronic health condition, high bloodpressure, a history of circulatory problems, heart problems and even a high resting heart-beat.

Getting Going

Everyone needs some type of motivation to get going on an exercise program. You may be looking for slimmer thighs, a flatter tummy or an all-round feeling of good health. Exercise is a key element in a healthy life and if you've got your health, the sky is the limit of what you can achieve.

All you've got to do now is make a commitment to a regular exercise program. Once you've done this, just stand back and watch the emergence of your new body. You'll see the results staring back at you in the mirror, chubby thighs and bulging stomachs will melt away and you'll feel and look terrific.

'Sounds great' you say to yourself, 'but I don't have the time . . . I'm too out of shape . . . I'm naturally heavy . . . and so forth. The mind loves to put up barriers but below we have provided a few tricks which will help you to get around your mind's protests.

1) Make your exercise period **your own special time** where you concern yourself only with your own body. Forget the stresses of job, family and friends and think of how beneficial these exercises are for your body's beautification and health.

2) **When to exercise.** Make exercise a part of your daily routine, whether in the early morning, at lunch breaks or before supper, whenever suits you best. Remember this is your time to get away from it all.

3) **Where to exercise.** Choose a spot that makes you feel good and relaxed, like your bedroom floor. All you need is some type of mat for the floor, a towel or blanket will do fine, and be sure to have enough space to kick your legs around. You can put little personal touches around you for inspiration, like a picture of yourself 20 lbs. lighter. And finally, use music. Put your favourite dynamic or soothing music on, and you'll find that the exercise time will fly by.

4) **What to wear.** Wear whatever makes you feel really comfortable. You don't have to buy special clothing but it is fun to have a specific outfit to wear that makes you feel good. Since you'll be stretching and toning muscles and working up a healthy perspiration, choose clothes that are easy to move in and easy to wash. If you like to feel professional about your work-out (another useful motivational tool) you can choose leotards and tights or a cheerful sweat suit, but anything non-constricting goes. The important thing is COMFORT.

5) **Results.** If you're an instant result seeker **don't** get on the scale. You're sure to see positive changes in a short while in terms of flexibility and tone. If you need measured results, use a tape measure once a week around the bulgy areas. In no time you'll be loosing inches. Look in the mirror after a few weeks and you'll find a noticeable difference.

A Reminder: Now that you're firming, toning and losing inches don't compensate with your eating habits. An added benefit of exercise is that it decreases appetite. Don't eat more because you're exercising more; maintain your present diet of moderation. Don't diet. Eat everything, but only have small portions of each.

Are you ready to get going? We hope so because the benefits you'll be reaping are just too good to pass up!

Rules of Yoga Practice

1) NEVER COMPARE YOURSELF TO ANYONE ELSE. Yoga emphasizes personal progress. Be careful not to go beyond the limit of your capability. By performing the exercise regularly you are bound to do better today than you did yesterday. In Yoga there is visible progress. You will find that after a relatively short time you will be able to get into more advanced poses without any danger of strain.

2) NEVER HURRY. Go into the postures slowly, taking ten to fifteen seconds to get from the beginning to the holding position. This gives bonus benefits, makes each exercise more effective and prevents injury.

3) HOLD EACH POSITION after you have gone as far into it as comfort permits. Muscles must undergo sustained effort in order to stay in condition. As a beginner, hold each posture at its extremity for five seconds. Increase this time by five seconds a week as you improve. Through the holding position you are doing an exercise over and over, as it were, and therefore an exercise need be repeated only three times, instead of twenty.

4) BREATHE NORMALLY during the holding position of an exercise. There is a tendency for most people to hold their breath while they desperately and tensely hold on. This is absolutely wrong. Yoga stresses relaxation, even while exercising. You should go as far into a pose as comfort permits, then relax there and breathe as normally as comfort permits. As a student advances in proficiency there is a prescribed way of breathing with each exercise. Generally speaking, one should exhale when going into a pose and inhale as one comes out of it. The notable exception is the Locust.

5) NEVER FORCE A POSITION. Never jerk or bounce in order to 'go further'. Go as far as you can, then hold it there. Pain is a danger signal devised by the body to stop immediately or risk injury. If, as in calisthenics, you are moving so fast that your momentum does not permit you to stop short, you can easily move past the danger signal and get hurt. This is what has happened when you experience muscular soreness or muscle strain.

6) CONCENTRATE INTENSELY with each exercise you perform. This is especially necessary in balancing exercises. Avoid moving your head rapidly, speaking or laughing selfconsciously when you exercise. Visualizing encourages concentration which, in turn, promotes quality of action. Also it will make exercising more fun.

7) COME OUT OF AN EXERCISE AS SLOWLY, as you went into it. Not only do you lose at least a third of the value if you permit yourself to collapse, but you might even risk injury.

8) REST BETWEEN EXERCISES. The beauty of yoga lies in its gentleness. You need never experience draining fatigue or painful, sore muscles. Catch your breath, let the muscles rebound from a delightful stretch and permit the body to assimilate what it has learned.

9) ALWAYS KEEP YOUR BODY RELAXED, even at

the apex of a position, except for those parts which are directly involved in the pose. The effort you are making should never be mirrored in a distorted face.

10) THE BEST TIME TO EXERCISE is either first thing in the morning or last thing at night. You may prefer a short period at each of these times; it depends on your particular need. In the morning the body is still stiff, but the exercises will help you to work better all day. In the evening the exercising comes more easily and refreshes and relaxes you for a good sleep. Learn to use exercises as energizers or relaxers throughout the day.

11) PRACTISE REGULARILY, even if you have time for only a few exercises on some days. Then, do only those poses that you know do you the most good. Make yoga as integral to your daily routine as eating and sleeping. You will notice that the new strength and flexibility of your body will give you new vitality in your daily routine.

12) GOOD POSTURE usually means good health. Strive to maintain your body in its normal position. Military standards for good posture may help you to improve yours. Tuck the bottom in and imagine that someone is gently pulling you up by the hair of your crown.

13) EXERCISING ON AN EMPTY STOMACH will make your exercising period more comfortable. Try to exercise at least an hour and a half after meals. You'll be less susceptible to discomfort and that bloated feeling.

14) LASTLY, HAVE FUN. Yoga is good for your body and you can enjoy the fact that your body is getting in better shape with every exercise you do.

Kareen's Very Own Schedule

(age 42)

I. Warm-ups (p. 20)

II. One of these Aerobic Activities:
  a) bouncing on mini-trampoline
  b) runing in place alternated with stair-stepping
  c) dancing to vigorous music
  d) walking fast up a steep hill alternated with swimming, bicycling, skiing, in season.

III. Yoga Schedule
  a) Sun Salutations (3)
  b) Abdominal Lift (3)
  c) Triangle Poses
  d) Spread Leg Stretch — Standing
  e) Locust and Bow on alternate days
  f) Leg-Overs
  g) Sit-ups
  h) Twist
  i) Side Leg Lifts
  j) Plough & Shoulderstand — Alt.
  k) Crossed-Knee Bend
  l) Digestive Cycle

My problem areas are the tummy & thighs therefore I included b), e), f), g), h), i), and j) for the former and a), c), d), f), g), i) for the latter.

I have never had problems with my hips, but for general fat loss I have to include lots of leg and buttocks exercises.

Carl's Very Own Schedule (age 53)

I. Warm-Ups

II. One of these Aerobic Activities:
   a) bouncing on mini-trampoline
   b) dancing to vigorous music
   c) fast, arm-swinging walk
   d) stair-climbing, alternated with swimming, canoeing, skating and cross-country skiing, in season.

III. Yoga Schedule
   a) Arm and Leg Stretch
   b) Locust
   c) Triangle
   d) Abdominal Lift
   e) Pump
   f) Sit-up
   g) Rockn' Rolls
   h) Chest Expander
   i) Cobra
   j) Catstretch
   k) Alternate Leg Stretch
   l) Digestive Cycle or Complete Breath

"My problem areas are the tummy and my flexibility. I like to exercise the large muscles of the leg and buttocks for caloric expenditure and strength.

On busy days, I may only use lots of stairs during the working day, and the mini-trampoline at night. On it, I run, twist and do different-level exercises. If I follow that with Sit-ups, I feel I have done my bit for the day.

Your Very Own Schedule

_____

_____

_____

_____

_____

_____

_____

_____

_____

_____

_____

_____

_____

_____

_____

_____

Your Very Own Schedule, Revised

_____

_____

_____

_____

_____

_____

_____

_____

_____

_____

_____

_____

_____

_____

YOGA EXERCISES

General Advice on Warming Up

Before you start exercising, you should give your body a chance to warm up in order to avoid injury. You may compare the process to warming up your car on a cold morning. No mechanic would dream of racing the motor right away. You want to get the circulation going and to stretch tense muscles gently. There is no mystique to this, it can be done in a variety of ways.

You may of course, use such tried and true Yoga warm-ups as the Rock'n Rolls, but you can also do it just by getting the body moving. Stand there, take a few relaxing breaths and start:

Rolling	Hanging loose, like a rag doll
Shivering	Running-in-place
Shaking	Moving your body in rhythm to nice music
Stretching	Breathing Deeply
Bending	

Do not use music by the Bee Gees, the Supremes, Rod Stewart, The Rolling Stones, Paul McCartney & Wings, Janis Joplin and Jimi Hendrix, by the way. The beat in their music sounds like dit-dit-da, whereas the beat of the heart is da-dit and the beat of the blood vessels is da-dit-dit. In other words, these particular rock beats are opposite to the beat of the heart and therefore cause us stress. Since we constantly monitor our heart beat we subconsciously feel that something must have gone wrong when we hear another beat.

I remember once dancing vigorously to the Saturday Night Fever record of the Bee Gees and collapsing in an exhausted heap, convinced I was going to have a heart attack. Now I know that it was the beat that did me in, not the dancing — a most desirable aerobic activity. Classical music such as waltzes, popular tunes and oddly enough, Elvis records are fine, however.

Please do not underestimate the importance of warming-up. Muscle cells are the only part of the body that can increase their energy by up to 50 times, in a split second. All cells in the body need energy, of course, but only the muscles need so much so quickly for sudden bursts of activity, for 'springing into action'. If the muscle is totally 'cold' it is much more 'brittle' and vulnerable to injury. Warmed-up, it can do its work to make you look taut, smooth and trim much more efficiently.

Three-in-One Powerhouse Exercises

To Reduce Hips, Tummy and Legs

If you give me a choice of an exercise just for my tummy and an exercise that is good for my tummy, my waist and my legs all at the same time, I'll choose the 3-in-1 exercise every time. Who wouldn't? It's just plain good economy. That is why we have given you the following work-out. It applies equally to men and women and saves you a lot of effort and time, through triple benefits.

Of course, it is impossible to exercise just a tummy and not involve other muscles and organs to some degree. What makes our exercises special is that they are equally as powerful in all three areas. Abdominal exercises could be said to be dividable into two distinct areas: the upper abdomen and the lower abdomen. Men seem to get fat in the upper area, women in the lower. We have taken that into consideration in our planning and made the 3-in-1 Powerhouse Exercises general, whereas the 2-in-1 exercises are specific to the sexes. You see, if you have a fat tummy, there will always be a waist involvement. Hence you would be well advised to include some of the 3-in-1's (whichever you seem to need most and which seem to do most for you) in your schedule and then add the 2-in-1's that are relative to your sex.

You may wonder why we have included leg exercises in our 3-in-1's. What have legs to do with waist and abdomen? Nothing, but they do have a lot to do with reducing **general** fat in the body (see introductory article, p.22). Since the leg and buttocks muscles are the largest in the body, they need the most energy in being exercised and therefore they burn up the greatest number of calories! To lose fat in the waist, exercise the legs! It will make you a better athlete, too. Leg-exercises are excellent for such sports as skiing, tennis and racquet ball. For your easier reference, the exercises are arranged alphabetically. Make up your own schedule by which exercises seem the most challenging ones for you, not by how easy they are. The more you seem to have to work on a certain exercise, the more you probably need it.

Arm & Leg Stretch

Waist
Tummy
Legs

Stand straight, heels
together, toes pointing
slightly outward. Raise
right arm slowly at
an angle till hand is
above head, elbows
are straight.
Bend left knee and
bring leg close to
buttocks, shifting body
weight onto pelvis and
right foot. Grasp left
foot with left hand.

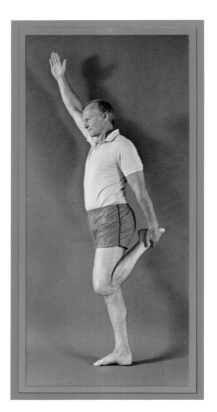

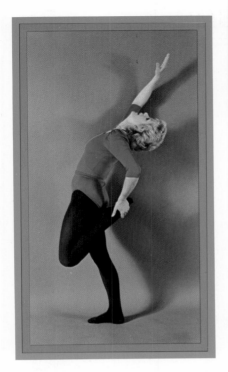

Exhale. Bend backward from the waist, pulling on left foot and moving right arm as far back as possible, head drops back. Hold 5 seconds. Repeat 3 times on both sides.

Remember to:

■ Try simpler balancing exercises at first.

■ Concentrate and your balance will be better.

Bow

Waist
Tummy
Hips

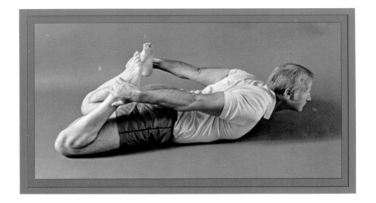

Lie on your tummy.
Bend your knees and
bring them close to
the buttocks.

Grasp your ankles
tightly. Lift head.
Inhale. If you have
difficulties, hold only
one ankle at a time.

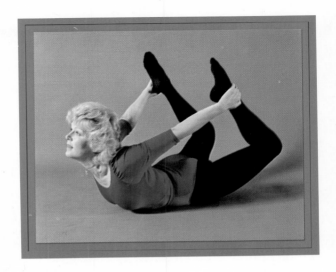

Exhale and lift your knees off the floor by pushing against your hands in an away motion. Hold 5 seconds or more. Repeat 3 times.

Remember to:

■ Push away from hands rather than pulling up to get knees off the floor.

■ Come out of the position slowly. Do not collapse.

Variations

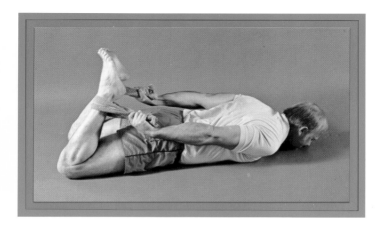

Use a towel or scarf around the ankles, if you cannot reach them with your hands.

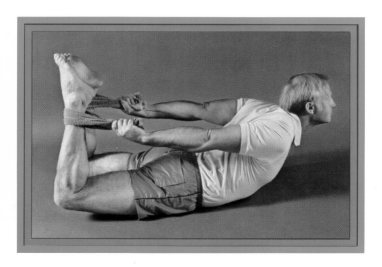

Push away from hands rather than pulling up to get knees off the floor.

Leg-Over

Waist
Tummy
Legs

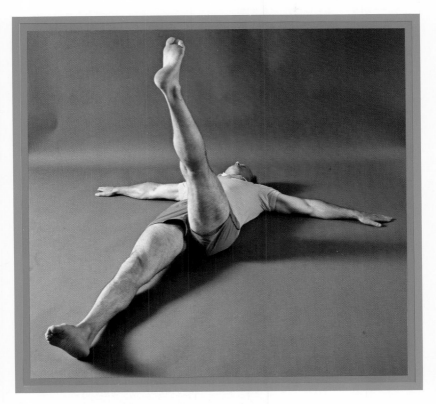

Lie on your back, arms outstretched.

Inhale and lift left leg straight up.

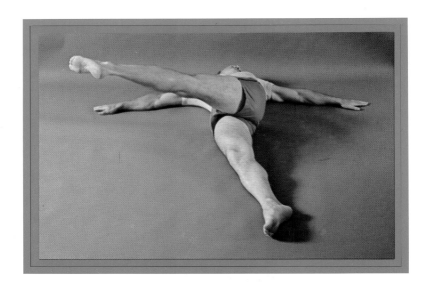

Now exhale and lower leg across the body to the left. Try to touch floor.
Keep both shoulders on the floor, turn head in opposite direction and hold pose for 5 seconds or longer. Repeat sequence twice more.

Remember to:

■ Keep leg straight throughout.

■ Keep **both** shoulders on the floor.

■ Put leg on a chair if you are out of shape or elderly.

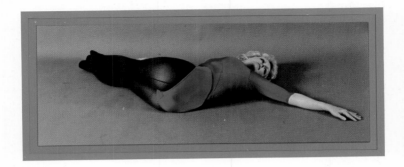

Lie with the legs straight up. Breathe in and
bring both legs down on the side as you exhale.
Try to touch the floor and hold for 5 seconds.

Locust

Waist
Tummy
Legs

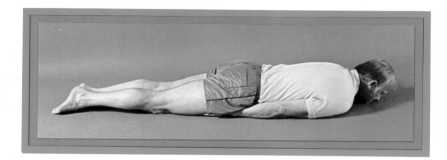

Lie on tummy, chin
against floor. Arms
are by your sides and
palms under thighs.

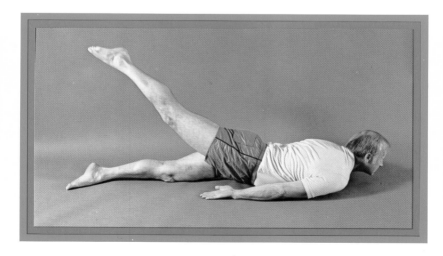

Inhale, lift head and
left leg as high as
they will go.

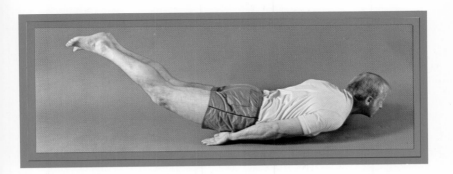

Hold pose and breathe
for 5 seconds. Chin
on floor. Exhale and
lower body slowly.

Repeat with other leg.
Eventually you can
lift both legs.

Remember to:

■ Push down on hands to get legs higher.

■ Keep legs straight.

■ Stiffen body as you thrust upward.

Variations

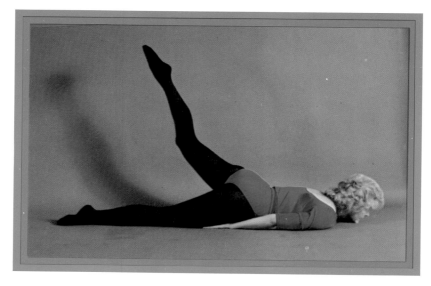

1 With legs raised as high as possible and arms folded in front of you, scissor-kick up and down 12 times.

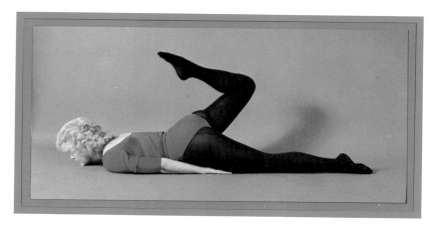

2 Raise one leg, then bend and straighten knee six times while leg stays up. Repeat on other side.

Side Raise

Waist
Tummy
Legs

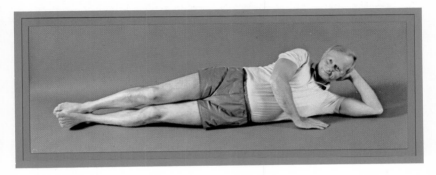

Lie on right side, right
arm outstretched, left
arm on floor in front
of chest. Inhale.

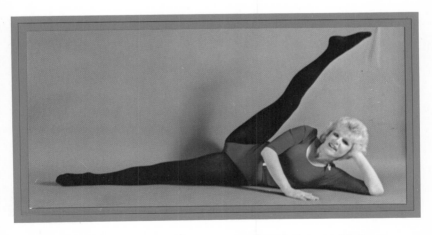

Keep the body in a
straight line. Exhale,
raise left leg as high
as it will go and hold
5 seconds.

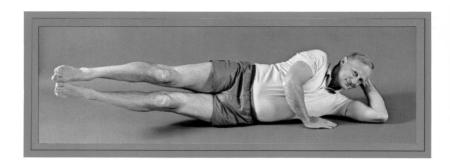

Lower leg slowly,
repeat twice more.

Repeat sequence on
other side.

Remember to:

■ Keep body straight, don't bend forward at waist.

■ Push down on hand in front of you, to get leg up higher.

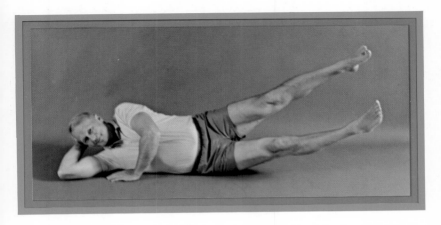

1 Lie on right side, supporting your weight on lower right arm. Raise one leg then bring the second up to meet the first. Repeat 3 times. Repeat on other side. Lower together.

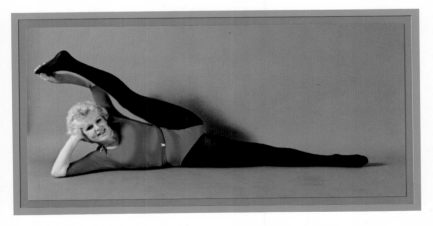

2 Lie on right side supporting your weight on lower right arm. Raise left leg as high as possible. Grasp toes with left hand. Repeat twice more. Repeat on other side.

Spread Leg Stretch Standing

Waist
Tummy
Leg

Stand with feet spread apart as far as possible.

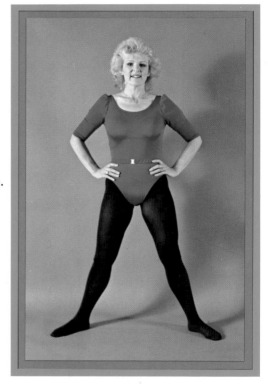

Remember to:

- Keep knees and back straight
- Keep the head, hands and legs all in a straight line.

Bend forward
and place hands on
floor. Inhale, bring
head up.

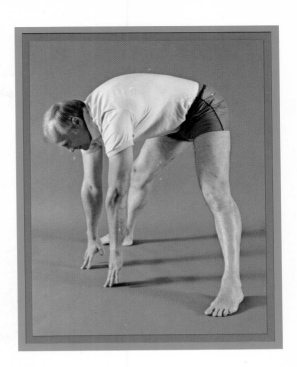

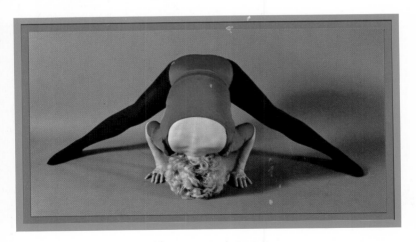

Exhale, bend elbows
and try to place top of
head on the floor.

Hold pose, breath
normally. Exhale and
straighten up. Repeat
twice more.

Staff

Waist Tummy Legs

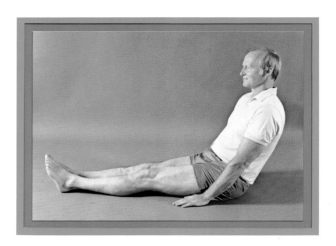

Sit on your tailbone, on the floor, with legs outstretched and arms by hips.

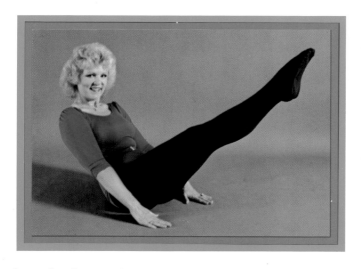

Lean back, exhale. Slowly raise legs to head level.

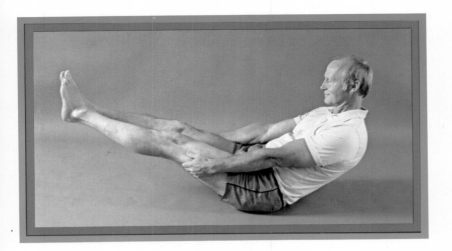

Hold as long as you can, breathe normally. Lower slowly and repeat 2 times more.

Exhale, lift legs and support them by holding along bottom of thighs. Hold. Lower. Repeat.

Remember to:

■ Concentrate intensely. Essential for a balancing pose.

■ Get your balance by lifting feet an inch or two at first. Then move very slowly.

■ Try again if you roll over on your back. Everyone does it at first.

Variations

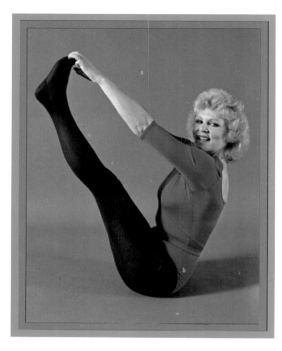

1

Sit as above. Bend knees, grab ahold of toes, lift heels and lean back to get your balance. Slowly straighten knees, hold.

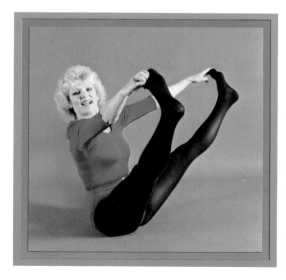

2

Sit as above. Bend knees, grab ahold of toes, lift heels and lean back. Straighten knees and slowly spread legs apart as far as they will go. Hold. Repeat.

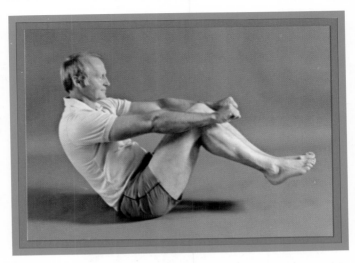

3 Rowboat: Sit with your knees slightly bent and arms outstretched.For fun do the exercise together with a friend. Bend forward as though to pull on oars,

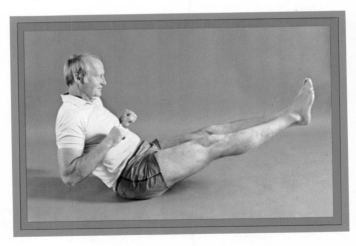

then lean back, lifting the legs and bringing fists to chest. Repeat ten to twenty times.

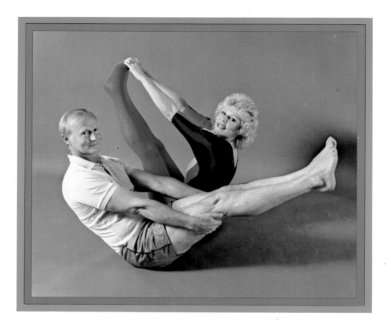

4 For fun do the exercises with a partner.

Sun Salutations

Waist
Tummy
Legs

Stand with the feet
slightly apart, the
hands together in front
of the chest.

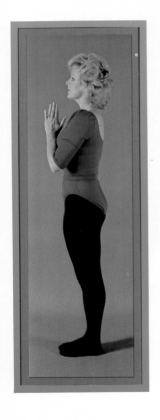

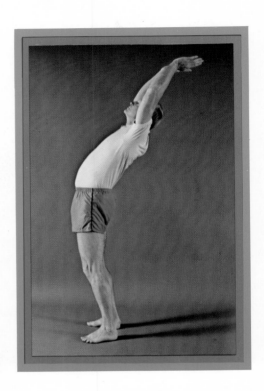

Inhale, raise the arms
over the head and
bend slowly backwards
from the waist,
pushing the pelvis
forward.

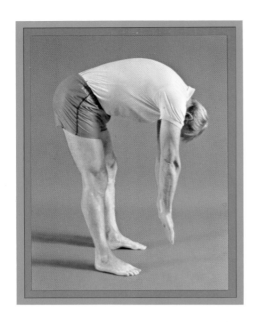

Exhale, bend forward and bring the hands to the floor beside the feet, knees straight.

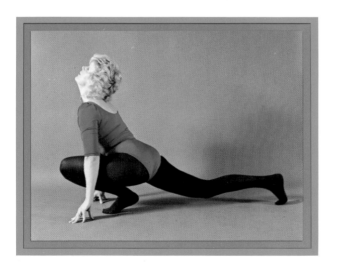

Inhale, bend the knees and bring the right foot back, resting the left thigh on the calf. Keep the bottom down, keep the right knee straight, raise the head and try to arch the back.

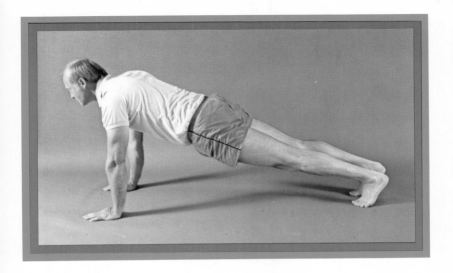

Hold the breath and bring the left leg alongside the right one, keeping the body in a straight line, with only the hands and toes supporting the body.

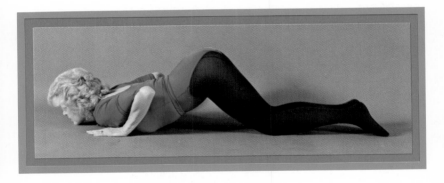

Exhale and slowly lower the body to the floor in this order: knees, forehead and chest.

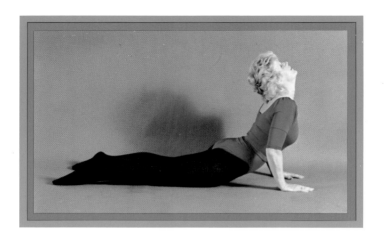

Inhale and in a smooth motion lower the pelvis to the floor, at the same time raising the head and arching the back in a Cobra position.

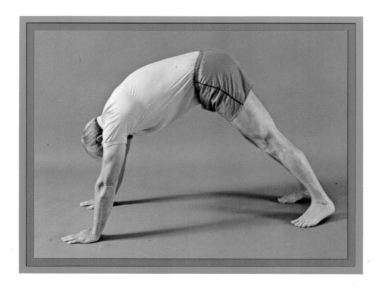

Exhale, push down on the hands, stick the bottom up, straightening the knees, and push down on the heels.

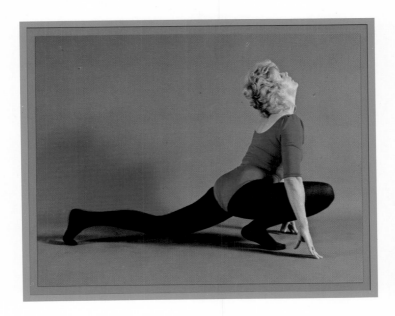

Inhale and bring the right foot forward setting it down between the hands. Keep the left leg extended, raise the head and arch the back.

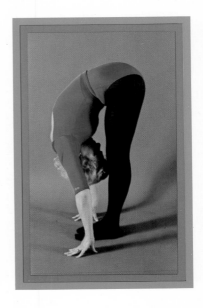

Exhale, bring the left leg forward, straighten the knees and perform a Forward Bend, the head as close to the knees as possible.

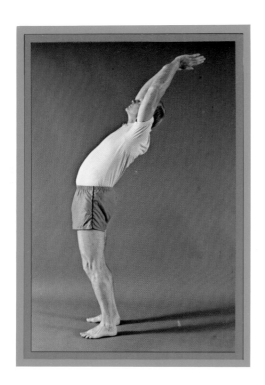

Inhale, straighten up with the arms over the head and bend back again as far as you can go.

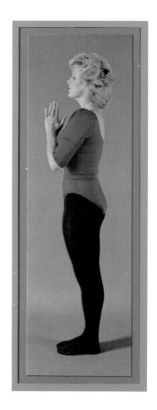

Exhale, come forward, lower the arms and relax.
Repeat this cycle once more in smooth fluid motions, eventually working up to 12 repetitions.

Remember to:

■ Pause for a moment, rather than hold.

■ Concentrate on the proper breathing technique.

■ Straighten the outstretched leg, but keep the knees and the tucked under toes touching the floor.

■ Do raise the head and arch the back. This means the bottom is tucked in.

Triangle Pose

Waist
Tummy
Legs

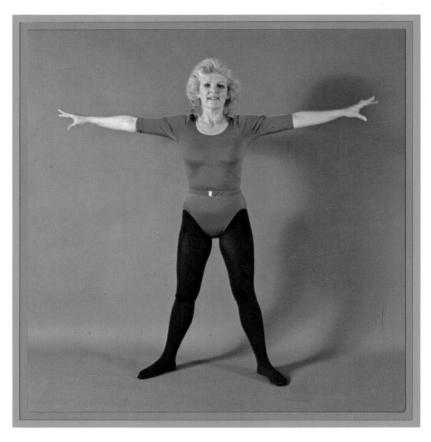

Stand with feet 3 feet apart. Bring arms out straight at sides. Point right foot far right, left foot slightly right.

Bend body to the right and bring right hand as close as possible to the outside of right foot.

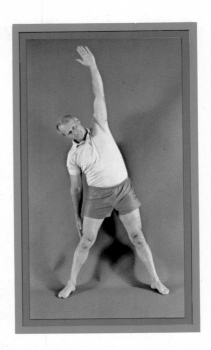

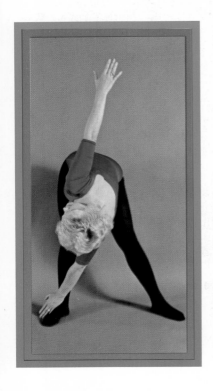

Move left arm up until it is in straight line with right arm. Look up at left hand. Hold 10 - 30 seconds. Repeat 2 times more on each side.

Remember to:

■ Keep both knees straight throughout.

■ Stretch shoulders as you hold.

Variations

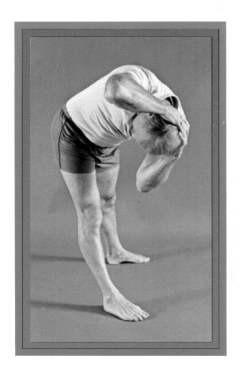

With arms clasped behind head, bend forward and bring elbow close to opposite knee. Repeat on the other side. Repeat twice more on each side.

Two-In-One Exercises For Men To Reduce the Waist & Tummy

Because men are rarely interested in hip exercises and women are desperately so, we have divided the poses that have two distinct benefits into sections for men and women. The men's section puts emphasis on the upper abdomen and waist, the women's is separated into two sections. One concentrates on the lower abdomen and the hips. The other offers poses that combine benefits from the waist and the hips.

Of course, poses are basically unisex and there are no undesirable side-effects if you particularily like a pose from the other section! The poses are particularily powerful for their specific areas and are highly recommended if you have bulges there. Spot-reducing fat is virtually impossible, but what is possible is to help the squat, fat-laden muscles regain their lean and slinky look by stretching them.

In this way you are toning and firming the offending areas as general body fat is being lost by a combination of diet, cardiovascular (or aerobic) exercise and yoga. As muscles flatten out, you will look considerably slimmer and will be able to fit into a size eight dress rather than a twelve. All this, without weight loss, because muscles weigh considerably more than fat. As you are changing the fat back into muscle through exercise, you are actually losing 'weight', but gaining muscle. Men have been known to change from a size 40 to a size 34 and even gain six or seven pounds. Yoga exercises help to make these metabolic changes in the muscles as they stretch them and keep you supple and therefore relaxed.

Abdominal Lift

Waist
Tummy

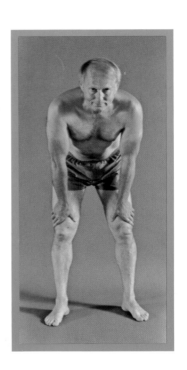

Stand slightly bent
forward, hands on
knees, knees bent
and a foot apart. Shift
your weight fully onto
knees, elbows straight.

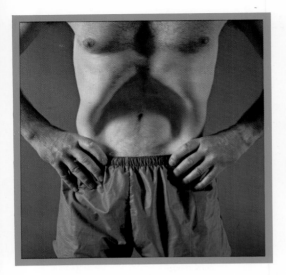

Inhale, then exhale completely and hold the exhalation **without breathing throughout the rest of the exercise.** Press chin against chest and pull tummy in as far as it will go. Hold for as long as you can. Now bang tummy out, inhale deeply and stand up.

Remember to:

■ Make sure your lungs are completely empty when you pull your abdomen in.

■ Relax as much as possible in the pose.

■ Keep practicing if you can't get a hollow and a ridge at first. It will come.

Variations

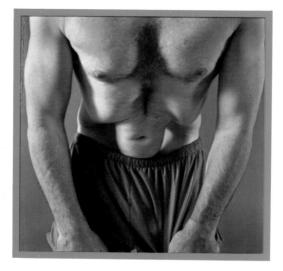

1 As above, but bang tummy in and out several times without holding in between, but without breathing — **on the exhalation.**

2 As above but after exhaling completely expand the chest and push the tummy out in a ridge.

The Pump

Waist
Tummy

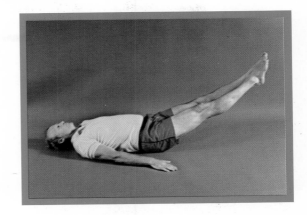

Lie on back with
outstretched legs, arms
by your side and
palms down. Push
down on palms, exhale
slowly and raise
straight legs to an
angle of 30°.

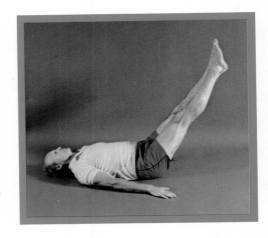

Hold for awhile. Exhale
and raise to a 60°
angle.

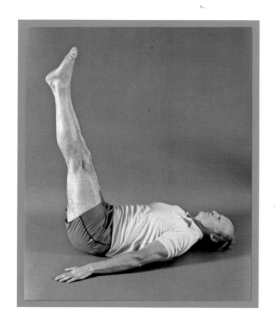

Hold, exhale and lift legs straight up to a 90° angle. Hold. Exhale, lower legs slowly, slowing further as your legs approach the floor. Repeat twice more.

Remember to:

■ Do this pose very slowly to receive the greatest benefits.

■ Avoid bending your knees or lifting your head as you come out of the pose.

■ Breathe normally.

1

Bicycling. Lie on back, arms above head, one knee bent and lift the other off the floor. Bicycle slowly 4 to 6 times, keeping small of back firmly on the floor.

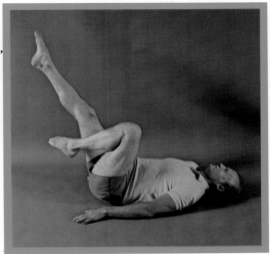

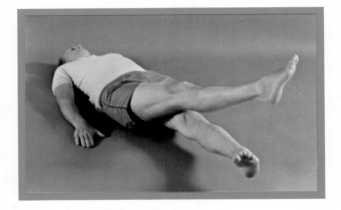

2 Scissors. Lie on back, hands under buttocks, legs extended two feet above floor. Lift head and criss-cross legs, opening them as wide as possible between 'scissors'. Repeat 15 - 25 times. Relax.

73

Sit-Up/Lie-Down

Waist
Tummy

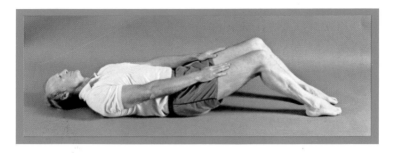

Lie on back, with knees bent so that foot is flat
on floor. Place hands flat on thighs.

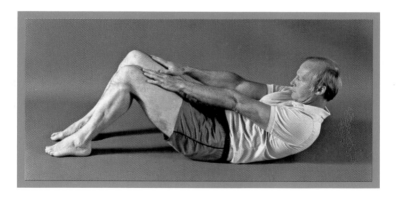

Lift head slowly, raising upper body to a 30
degree angle off of floor. Hands slide up legs till
fingertips brush knee-caps. Keep back straight and
hold 5 - 10 seconds. Lower back and slowly
repeat 3 - 5 times.

Remember to:

■ Put more emphasis on lying down than sitting up.

■ Stay at a 30 degree angle.

■ Breathe normally throughout.

■ Always tighten tummy muscles before you go into the pose.

Variations

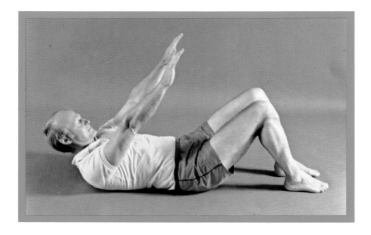

1 Lie on back, knees bent, arms extended above head. Swing arms forward as you sit up and extend legs. Hold. Lower slowly. Repeat 5 times.

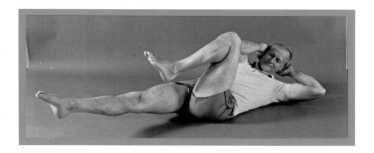

2 Lie on back, knees close to chest. Tighten tummy muscles and with hands clasped behind head, bring right elbow to left knee and extend right leg. Repeat on other side in a bicycling fashion. Repeat whole sequence at least twice more.

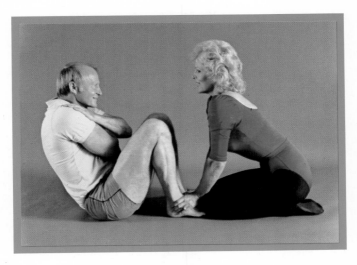

3 Sit as close to heels as possible, hands crossed on chest. Have a partner hold your feet down or place them under the couch.

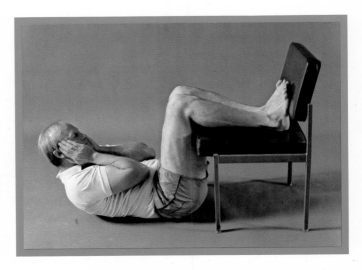

4 Lie flat on your back, legs up on a chair, hands on chin. Tense tummy muscles and lift head and chest as far as they will go. Lower. Repeat 3-12 times.

Trunk Sealer

Waist
Tummy

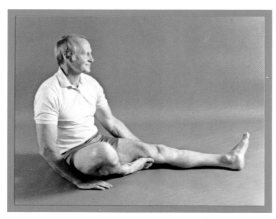

Sit with legs outstretched and slightly apart.
Bend left knee till the sole of the foot is right
against right thigh.

Exhale, bend forward and grab right big toes with
both hands. Pull chin in tightly against chest.
Stretch back up, shoulders rounded.

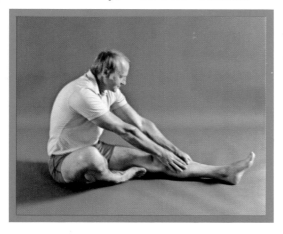

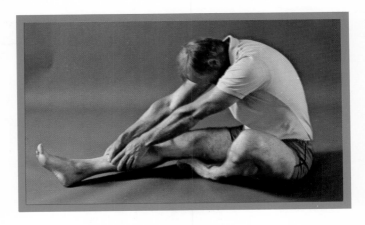

Inhale, pulling abdomen in sharply in a whacking motion. Exhale, pushing tummy out. Inhale, tightening abdomen again, etc. Repeat to 2 minute duration.

Remember to:

- Press head to chest
- Keep spine stretched upwards.
- Keep right leg straight and toes tightened.

Ear to Knee Pose

Waist
Tummy

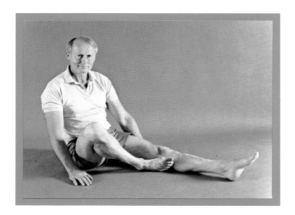

Sit, legs outstretched and apart. Bend left leg and bring foot against right thigh. Knee falls to one side.

Place right lower arm palm-up on right thigh. Turn body left so it is at right angle to right leg. Raise left arm and bring over hand.

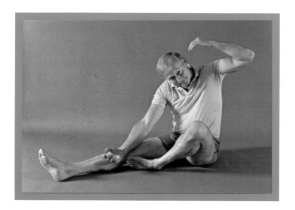

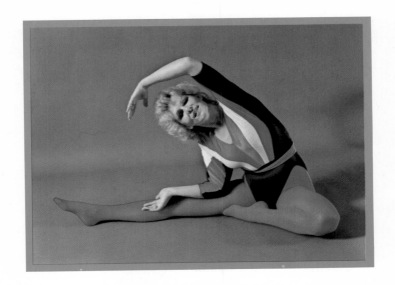

Exhale. Bend to the right and grasp inside arch of right foot with right hand. Left hand grasps the same foot from the outside. Point face towards front, the ear against right knee. Hold 5 - 20 seconds. Repeat on other side.

Remember to:

■ Keep palm upward.
■ Keep knee straight.
■ Twist body forward and up for extra benefits.

Two-In-One Exercises For Women To Reduce Tummy, Hips and Legs

Cat Stretch

Tummy
Hips
Waist

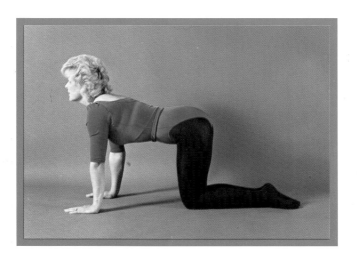

Kneel on all fours.

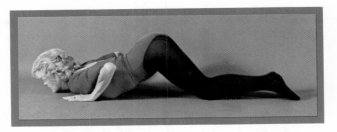

Rock backward and lower chest in a foreward sweeping motion. Hold 5 seconds. Return to original position.

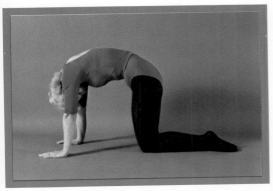

Arch back upward as far as possible. Hold 5 seconds and relax. Repeat twice more.

Remember to:

- Move slowly and with grace. Enjoy the stretch.

- Don't get discouraged if the leg is far away from head. It comes with practise.

83

Variations

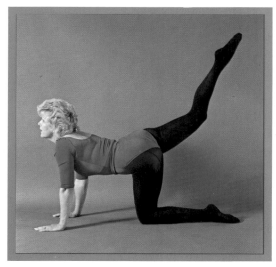

Kneel on all fours, extend one leg out in back and swing it forward. Repeat several times slowly. Repeat on other side.

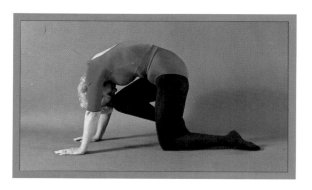

As above, but swing leg out to side and describe little circles with it. Circle 5 times clockwise, five times counterclockwise.

Deep Lunge

Tummy
Hips
Legs

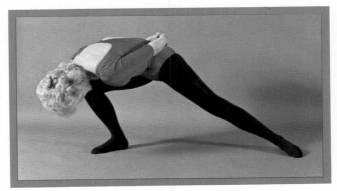

Stand with feet apart. Turn the right foot to a 90 degree angle to body, left foot points forward. Bend right knee, exhale and clasp hands behind back. Bend body forward, resting chest on right thigh.

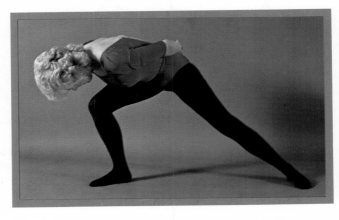

At same time, slide left leg back as far as possible, keeping knee straight.

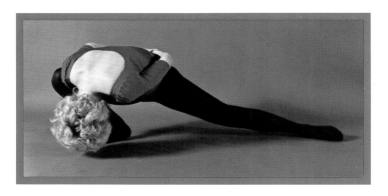

After establishing balance, slowly slide chest off inside thigh and attempt to bring the head to the floor. Hold 10 - 30 seconds. Exhale, straighten up. Repeat on other side.

Remember to:

- Point left foot forward for better balance.

- Use hands as a support in the beginning.

- Use body weight to bring head to floor rather than bouncing.

- Keep left knee straight.

Knee Press

Tummy
Hips
Waist

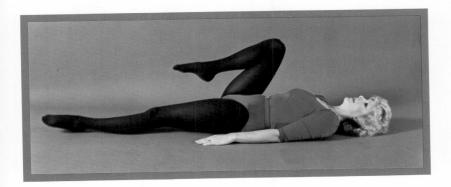

Lie flat on back with legs outstretched and
hands at sides. Bend right knee and bring up
against chest.

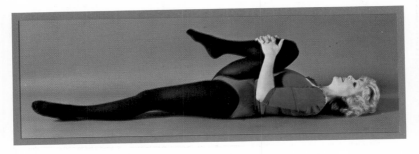

Inhale. With clasped hands press right knee
against chest and abdomen, leaving left leg
straight. Head does not lift off floor.
Hold pose and breathe for 5 - 10 seconds.
Repeat with other leg and both legs together.

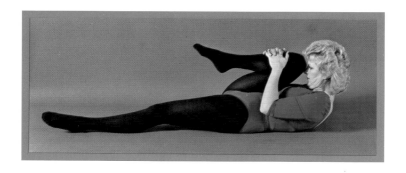

After bringing knee to chest, raise head and try to press forehead to knee. Hold 5 - 10 seconds. Repeat other leg.

Remember to:

■ Breathe if you have high blood pressure or heart trouble.

■ Get a good grasp of the knees and to exert maximum pressure on abdomen.

■ Remain encouraged. Beneficial whether head and knee touch or not.

1 Perform a situp with legs outstretched and hands on thighs. Inhale, and slowly lift head and shoulders as high as possible. Back remains on floor. Hold breath. Exhale and relax.

2 As above, with legs raised 3" off the ground.

3 As above, with hands clasped behind head.

Shooting Bow

Hips
Tummy
Waist

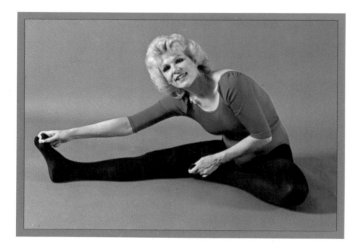

Sit on floor, legs
outstretched. Bend
forward and grasp right
big toe with right
hand, left toe with left
hand.

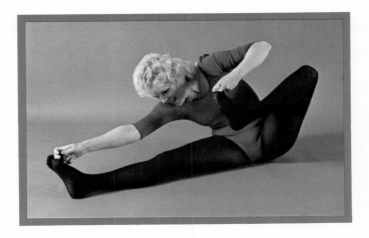

Exhale, bend right knee and pull right foot to right ear in one motion. Bring right shoulder back.

Keep hold of left leg, knee straight. Hold 5 -15 seconds. Repeat on other side.

Remember to:

- Keep outstretched leg on floor.
- Get a good grasp of ankles if you can't reach toes.
- Bend forward to meet foot at first then gradually straighten back.

Variations

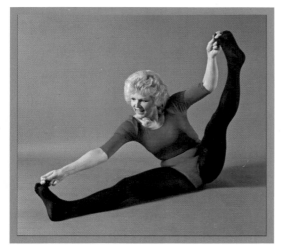

1

After holding pose, exhale and straighten right knee as far as you can. Hold 5 - 15 seconds. Relax.

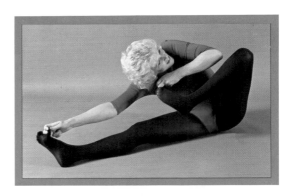

2 Pull right foot to left ear and hold.

Two-In-One Exercises For Women To Reduce Hips and Waist

Ankle to Forehead Stretch ▬▬▬

Hips
Waist

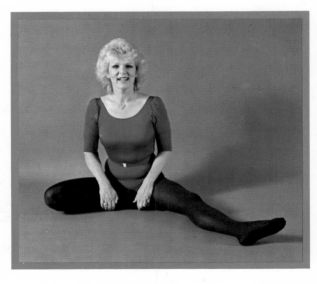

Sit with legs
outstretched. Bend right
leg and bring foot
close to the body,
knee to one side.

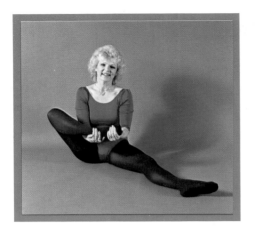

Grasp right foot from underneath at ankle with right hand. Left hand grasps ball of foot.

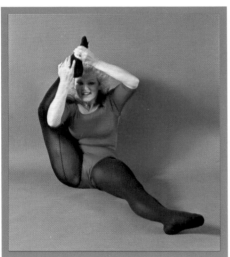

Bend head forward and pull ankle towards forehead. Hold 5 - 30 seconds, breathing normally. Repeat on other side.

Remember to:

■ Bend forward to get ankle and forehead together, straightening arms with improvement.

■ Keep opposite leg straight.

Inclined Plane ━━━━━━

Hips
Waist

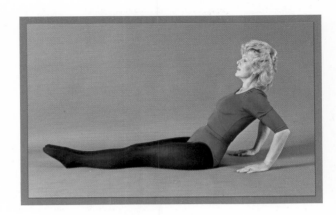

Sit, legs together and
outstretched. Lean
back slightly placing
hands straight down
from the shoulders,
fingers facing forwards.

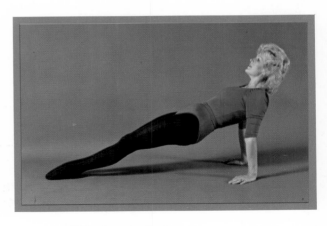

Exhale, push down
on hands and lift
buttocks off the floor.
Push hips up, arching
the back.

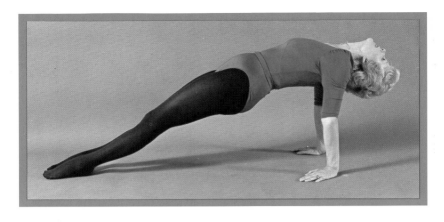

Let head fall back.
Hands and feet carry
body weight. Hold 10 -
60 seconds and lower
hips to floor. Relax.

Remember to:

■   Bend knees and have the soles of your feet flat
on floor to help with raising of buttocks at first.
Straighten as you get better.

■   Distribute body weight evenly between the hands
and feet.

■   Stretch neck back as far as possible when head is
hanging.

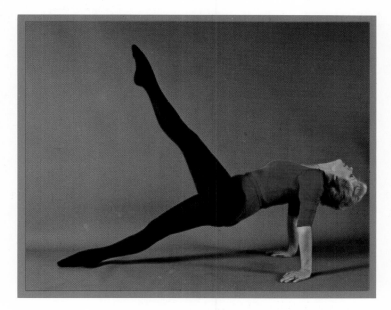

1 After back is arched, raise right leg slowly as high as possible.

Hold 10 - 30 seconds. Repeat other side.

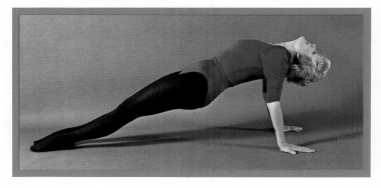

2 Legs as above but with fingers pointing hands are beside hips backwards.

Side Leg Lift

Hips
Waist

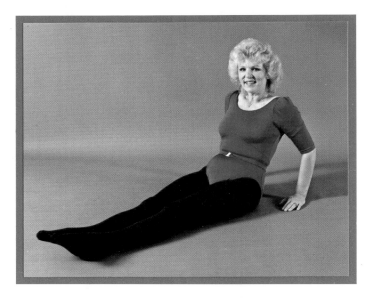

Sit, legs extended. Leaning back, place hands
straight down from shoulders, fingers pointing
towards sides.

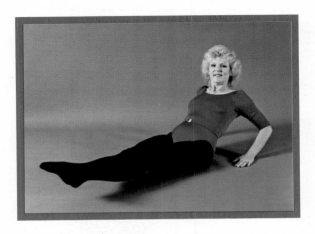

Bend elbows slightly and raise toes 3 inches
off ground.

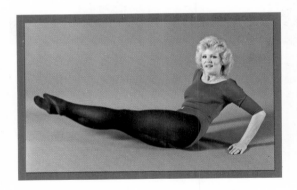

Move elevated legs slowly to the right
without raising. Go as far as possible, rolling
onto right hip.

Remember to:

- Keep a fairly upright position, elbows only slightly bent.

- Straighten right arm when legs are to the right and vice versa.

- Keep legs at the 3" level when crossing to side.
  As above, but raise legs as high as possible.

Variation

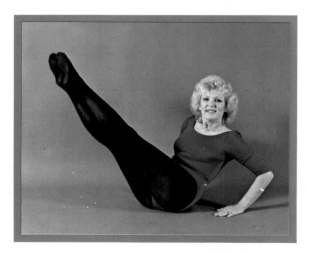

Exhale, lift legs as high as possible. Shift weight to the left and straighten right arm. Hold 3 - 4 seconds. Lower legs on side to 3" position. Bring legs forward and repeat on other side. Relax. Repeat sequence twice more.

As above, but perform exercise from one side to the other without stopping.

Reverse Arch

Hips
Waist

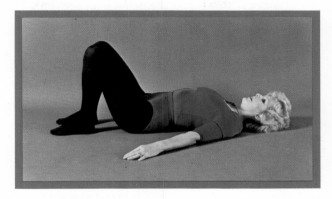

Lie on back, knees bent and arms by the sides.
Pull the feet as close to buttocks as possible.

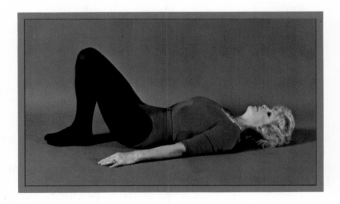

Exhale and slowly tilt pelvis upwards, pushing
small of back against floor. Hold pose and exhale.
Lower.

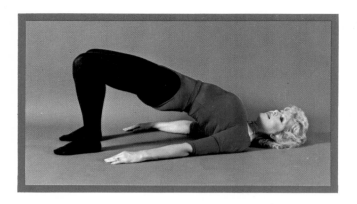

Inhale, slowly push buttocks and lower body as high as possible. Shift weight towards shoulders and breathe normally. Hold 5 - 10 seconds. Release slowly and repeat 3 - 4 times.

Remember to:

■ Tilt pelvis rather than lifting it. Buttocks are not wholly off the ground in second photo.

■ Keep weight on shoulders, not on arms.

The Twist

Hips
Waist

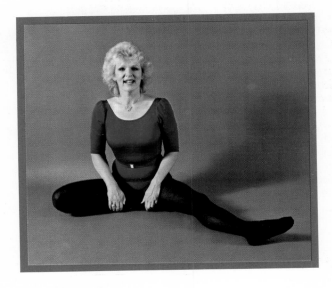

Sit on floor, legs
outstretched. Bend
right leg and bring
foot against left thigh.
Right knee presses
against floor.

Bend left leg and leave knee pointing up. Bring left foot over right knee and firmly plant it as far back as possible. Shift weight forward and using left hand as support, bring right arm between chest and left knee to floor. Twist your body so that the right shoulder rests against left knee, and push hard against the floor with your **left** hand, twisting to your left as much as you can. Turn head to left as though to peer over your left shoulder. Hold. Repeat in reverse on the other side.
Repeat each side twice more.

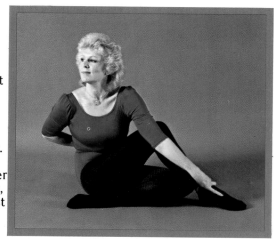

Remember to:

- Twist to the left if left knee is up and vice versa.
- Put your **right** arm between knee and chest if your **left** knee is up and vice versa.
- Push hand against the floor with your furthest arm to get a good twist.

Breaths For Men and Women

No Yoga book is ever complete without a chapter on breathing, nor should any exercise book be. After all, breath is life and oxygen is our most important 'food'. Too few know how to use this resource properly, however, and so they are considerably undernourishing themselves in energy. This is particularily relevant in this book where we talk about cardiovascular or aerobic exercises. The former means 'of the heart and blood vessels as a unified body system', the latter is derived from aerobiosis meaning 'life by means of air and oxygen'. Nowadays this generally refers to constant, steady exercise over a minimum of 15 minutes (at 80% of max.) to 45 minutes (at 70% of max.).

It becomes terribly important then, that you should know how to do properly, what you do so much of. Most people use only one-fifth of their potential in breathing. Imagine how much more vital and energetic you can feel by learning how to breathe well. Briefly, the diaphragm is a sheath of muscles separating the body into two cavities: the chest and the abdomen. The diaphragm is dome-shaped and presses against the bottom of the lungs. So, in order to fill the bottom of the lungs, you must flatten the diaphragm. As every singer knows, the only way you can do this is by pushing your tummy out. Contrary to everything you may ever have learned, you must push the tummy OUT as you INHALE, and pull the tummy IN when you EXHALE! This may be a little hard to remember in the beginning, but it easily becomes a habit with practise.

We know that deep breathing has an enormously relaxing and calming effect on the central nervous system. We know that the brain is a great consumer of oxygen and when its supply needs to be replenished, you have to yawn. We know that oxygen is very important in helping to burn off fat in the tissues. Surely, with such benefits, it makes excellent sense to 'invest' in good breathing habits.

Complete Breath

Sit in cross-legged position or in chair. Keep back straight. Slowly inhale deeply through nose. Take five seconds to fill lower lungs as you expand the abdomen and rib cage.

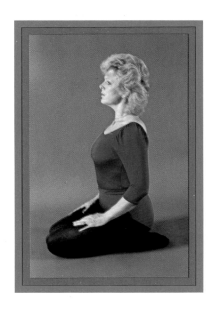

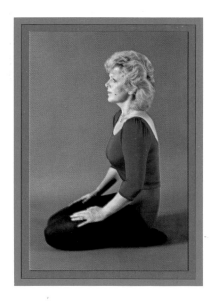

Fill middle and top of lungs for an additional 5 - 10 seconds, expanding chest. Hold 1 - 5 seconds. Exhale slowly. Repeat 4 - 5 times.

Remember to:

- Establish a rhythm in the rise and fall of the abdomen.

- Keep upright posture for maximum breathing efficiency.

- Push abdomen out on the in-breath and pull abdomen in on the out-breath.

- Imagine filling lungs like a coffee cup, bottom first.

Crossed Knee Bends

Stand, with spine erect.
Cross slightly bent
right knee over left.
Place toes next to
each other. Right
heel remains off floor.

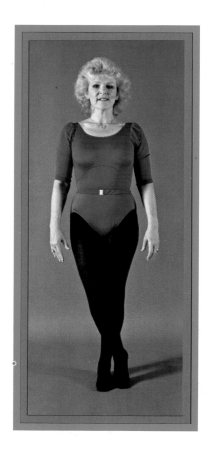

Inhale. Bend forward, keeping shoulders straight and spine centered. Exhale. Bring fingers as close as possible to floor. Let head hang loosely. Relax abdomen. Straighten gradually inhaling. Repeat each leg 3x.

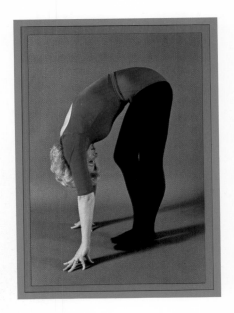

Remember to:

■   Keep spine centered. There is a tendency to favour one hip.

■   Bend from the waist and not from hips and shoulders.

■   Use a chair at first for confidence.

Digestive Cycle:
For better digestion:

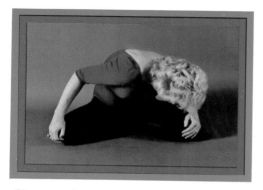

Sit, comfortably cross-legged, hands on knees.
Now describe a circle with your upper body in a
clockwise movement.

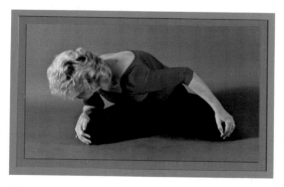

Lean back exhaling, pulling the abdomen IN,
then bend forward inhaling, pushing the abdomen
OUT.

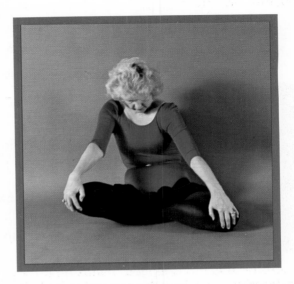

Repeat 4 times, then perform the same movement in an anti-clockwise direction. The rhythm is: bend forward — inhale — push tummy OUT: lean backward — exhale — pull tummy IN.

This is an easy, effective abdominal churning for the beginner and with the proper breathing, serves as a breath as well.

Remember to:

- Pull tummy in while exhaling.
- Push tummy out while inhaling.
- Do not practice with full stomach, while menstruating, pregnant or while suffering from ulcers.

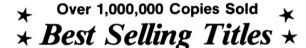